GET INFORMED—STAY INFORMED

UNIVERSAL
HEALTH CARE

Heather C. Hudak

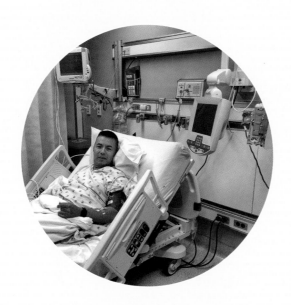

CRABTREE
PUBLISHING COMPANY
WWW.CRABTREEBOOKS.COM

Author: Heather C. Hudak
Series research and development:
Reagan Miller
Editor-in-chief: Lionel Bender
Editors: Simon Adams, Ellen Rodger
Proofreaders: Laura Booth,
Crystal Sikkens
Project coordinator: Melissa Boyce
Design and photo research:
Ben White
Production: Kim Richardson
Production coordinator and
Prepress technician: Margaret Amy Salter
Print coordinator: Katherine Berti
Consultant: Emily Drew,
Public Librarian, B.F.A., M.S.-LIS

Produced for Crabtree
Publishing Company by
Bender Richardson White

Photographs and reproductions: Alamy: 6 (dpa picture alliance), 8 (dong98), 10 (Jim West), 12 (Bastiaan Slabbers), 13 (Science History Images), 14–15 (Agencja Fotograficza Caro), 22–23 (B. Christopher), 26 top (Everett Collection), 32-33 (Ian Dagnell). Getty images: 20 (Barry Philp), 28–29 (Frederic J. Brown). Library of Congress: 17 (LC-USZC2-5334, WPA Federal Art Project). Shutterstock: heading band (deepadesigns), tablets icon (Oleksiy Mark), 1 (Casiohabib), 4 (Askolds Berovskis), 11 (Alexander Raths), 24–25 (Poznyakov), 26 bottom (Jeff Whyte), 30–31 (Alwin Lee), 33 (Monkey Business Images), 34 (VanderWolf Images), 35 (Rawpixel), 36–37 (Lesterfair), 38 (nitinut380), 39 (La Zona), 40–41 (GaudiLab), 43 (Heidi Besen). Topfoto: 16–17 (ullsteinbild), 18 (World History Archive), 19 (Granger NYC), 21 (Roger-Viollet).

Diagrams: Stefan Chabluk, using the following as sources of data: p. 7 OECD Health Data 2013/World Bank 2016. p. 18 World Bank and national statistics. p. 23 Huffington Post/GoBankingRates.com. p. 25 U.S. Institute for Health Metrics and Evaluation. p. 26 U.S. Congressional Budget Office. p. 29 U.S. Government statistics and OECD. p. 31 Bloomberg.com/Bay Area Council Economic Institute. p. 43 United Nations Department of Economic and Social Affairs

Library and Archives Canada Cataloguing in Publication

Title: Universal health care / Heather C. Hudak.
Names: Hudak, Heather C., 1975- author.
Series: Get informed--stay informed.
Description: Series statement: Get informed, stay informed |
Includes bibliographical references and index.
Identifiers: Canadiana (print) 20190241144 |
Canadiana (ebook) 20190241152 |
ISBN 9780778772750 (hardcover) |
ISBN 9780778772804 (softcover) |
ISBN 9781427124685 (HTML)
Subjects: LCSH: Medical policy—United States—Juvenile literature. |
LCSH: Medical care—United States—Juvenile literature. |
LCSH: Health services accessibility—United States—Juvenile
literature. | LCSH: Health care reform—United States—Juvenile
literature. | LCSH: National health services—Juvenile literature.
Classification: LCC RA395.A3 H83 2020 | DDC j362.10973—dc23

Library of Congress Cataloging-in-Publication Data

Names: Hudak, Heather C., 1975- author.
Title: Universal health care / Heather C. Hudak.
Other titles: Get informed--stay informed.
Description: New York, New York : Crabtree Publishing
Company, 2020. | Series: Get informed-stay informed |
Includes bibliographical references and index.
Identifiers: LCCN 2019054146 (print) | LCCN 2019054147 (ebook)
ISBN 9780778772750 (hardcover) |
ISBN 9780778772804 (paperback) | ISBN 9781427124685 (ebook)
Subjects: LCSH: Health insurance--United States--Juvenile
literature. | Health services accessibility--Economic aspects-
-United States--Juvenile literature. | Medical care, Cost
of--Juvenile literature. | Medical care--Finance--Government
policy--Juvenile literature. | Medical care--United States--
Juvenile literature. | Health care reform--Juvenile literature.
Classification: LCC RA412.2 .H83 2020 (print) |
LCC RA412.2 (ebook) | DDC 362.1/0425--dc23
LC record available at https://lccn.loc.gov/2019054146
LC ebook record available at https://lccn.loc.gov/2019054147

Crabtree Publishing Company

www.crabtreebooks.com   1-800-387-7650

Printed in the U.S.A./032020/CG20200127

Published in Canada
Crabtree Publishing
616 Welland Ave.
St. Catharines, ON
L2M 5V6

Published in the United States
Crabtree Publishing
PMB 59051
350 Fifth Avenue, 59th Floor
New York, NY 10118

Published in the United Kingdom
Crabtree Publishing
Maritime House
Basin Road North, Hove
BN41 1WR

Published in Australia
Crabtree Publishing
Unit 3 – 5 Currumbin
Court
Capalaba
QLD 4157

CONTENTS

1 A CONTROVERSIAL ISSUE

Imagine you broke your arm and needed a cast. Maybe your parents called an ambulance to take you to the hospital for treatment. These services cost money—often a lot. In some countries, people pay health expenses out of pocket or through private insurance. In others, a mixture of private insurance and public health care helps people pay health bills. In a universal health care system, everyone gets access to the health care they need when they need it, whether or not they can afford to pay.

I think ... [health care is] probably more of a privilege. Do you consider food a right? Do you consider clothing a right? Do you consider shelter a right? What we have as rights is life, liberty, and the pursuit of happiness. Past that point, we have the right to freedom. Past that point everything else is a limited resource that we have to use our opportunities given to us to afford those things. Wisconsin Republican Senator Ron Johnson's response to a high-school student who asked if he thought universal health care was a right, 2017

▶ An ambulance ride—as here in New York City, U.S.A.—is part of health care services and costs.

QUESTIONS TO ASK

Within this book are three types of boxes with questions to help your critical thinking about universal health care. The icons will help you identify them.

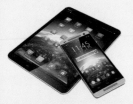

THE CENTRAL ISSUES
Learning about the main points of information.

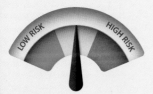

WHAT'S AT STAKE?
Helping you determine how the issue will affect you.

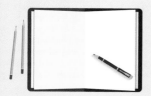

ASK YOUR OWN QUESTIONS
Prompts to address gaps in your understanding.

Health care is about more than just hospital visits. It includes all services needed to set up, maintain, and improve people's well-being throughout their entire lives. Among the services are medicines, doctor's examinations, disease prevention, and counseling. Universal health care programs aim to provide equal access to such services for everyone. They act as social insurance programs that follow the insurance model where risk is shared. People contribute to the insurance through taxes that the government uses to fund health care for all.

In other countries, people buy health insurance plans from the government or private companies. The money they pay for insurance, called **premiums**, is pooled into one big fund that is used to pay for the health services of anyone who needs them. Even if a person does not use health care, they must still pay their premiums. They are protected in case they need health care someday. Some countries use a combination of tax-funded and insurance programs, while other countries have hardly any health services at all.

UNDERSTANDING THE ISSUE

It is important to get informed about universal health care and the reasons why each country has chosen its model of health care. When people are misinformed about an issue, they often jump to inaccurate conclusions. Equipped with good information, and knowing how to use it, will help you understand the world around you and how such aspects of **society** impact your own life.

According to the World Health Organization (WHO), universal health care is an essential, fundamental **human right**. Most developed nations agree with the WHO, and offer all people access to the health services they need. They do not limit access to only those who can afford to pay for them. Many other countries are taking steps to achieve universal health care for all by 2030.

The United States is the only **industrialized** country in the world without some form of universal health care. Instead, people must purchase a private insurance plan, pay for

> " If your baby is going to die and it doesn't have to, it shouldn't matter how much money you make. I think that's something that whether you're a Republican or a Democrat or something else, we all agree on that, right? "
>
> U.S. comedian and talk show host Jimmy Kimmel's thoughts on his son's heart condition and the need for affordable health care in May 2017

▼ People rallied in Washington, D.C., on April 10, 2019, in support of Medicare, a U.S. government-funded health care program that provided coverage and long-term care for all U.S. citizens.

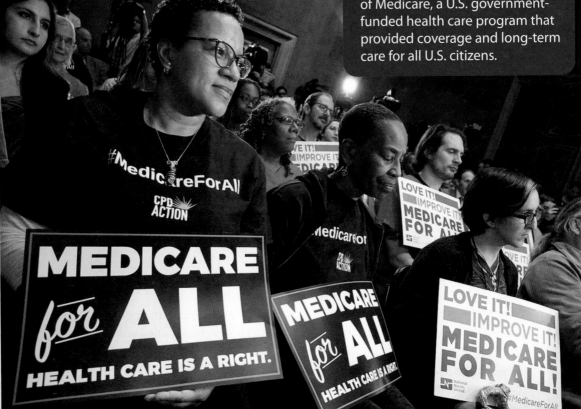

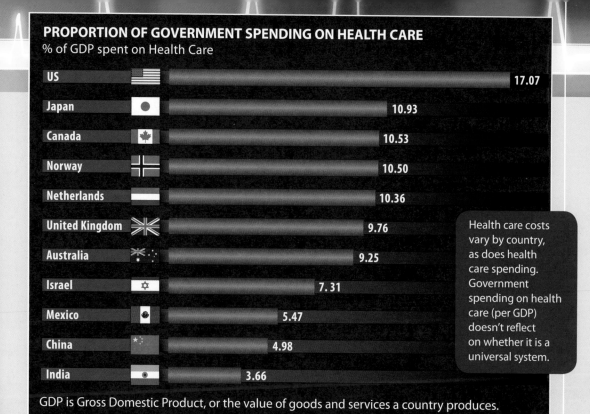

PROPORTION OF GOVERNMENT SPENDING ON HEALTH CARE
% of GDP spent on Health Care

Country	% of GDP
US	17.07
Japan	10.93
Canada	10.53
Norway	10.50
Netherlands	10.36
United Kingdom	9.76
Australia	9.25
Israel	7.31
Mexico	5.47
China	4.98
India	3.66

Health care costs vary by country, as does health care spending. Government spending on health care (per GDP) doesn't reflect on whether it is a universal system.

GDP is Gross Domestic Product, or the value of goods and services a country produces.

health care out of their own pockets, or qualify for a government support program. Private health insurance is a huge business in the United States. The system has been in place for a long time and would be hard to remove. Installing a new system would have a big impact on U.S. society as a whole.

A CONSTANT DEBATE

Regardless of the health care system each country has, governments everywhere face rising health care costs and need to find ways to deal with them. A growing population, care of the elderly, increased staff costs, and maintaining hospitals all play a part. Their governments constantly debate the pros and cons of each health care system and which one is right for them.

Canada has a universal health care system, but many people want to see improved and expanded health care services. Some even call for access to more private health care options. The reality is that health care providers face cuts in funding and services each year.

Because universal health care is always in the spotlight, you need to find out how to track its changes.

THE CENTRAL ISSUES

What are some of the benefits of tax-funded or affordable health care in the United States? What are some of the problems a universal health care program might create for U.S. citizens?

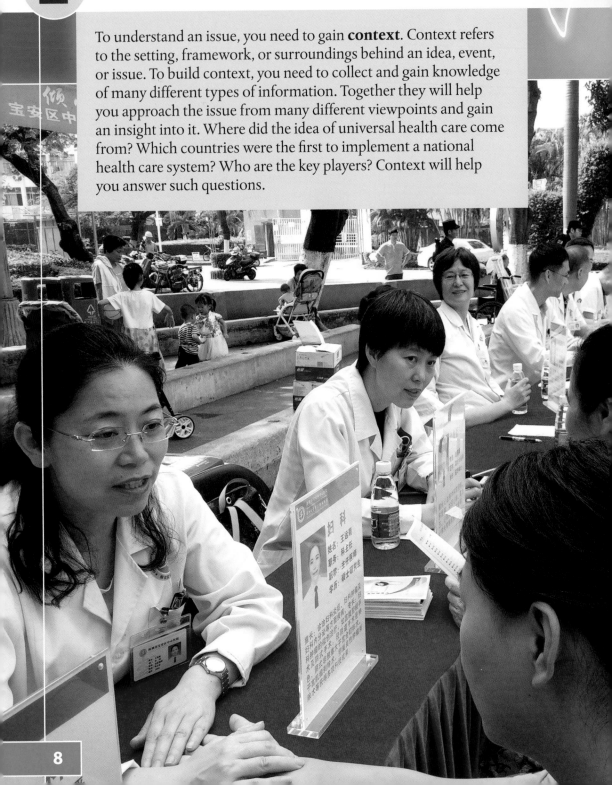

2

HOW TO GET INFORMED

To understand an issue, you need to gain **context**. Context refers to the setting, framework, or surroundings behind an idea, event, or issue. To build context, you need to collect and gain knowledge of many different types of information. Together they will help you approach the issue from many different viewpoints and gain an insight into it. Where did the idea of universal health care come from? Which countries were the first to implement a national health care system? Who are the key players? Context will help you answer such questions.

Medicare is a term countries such as Canada and Australia use for their **publicly funded** health care programs. In the United States, it refers to a federal health insurance program for the elderly and disabled.

In a **single-payer health care system** taxes are used to fund basic health services for all people at no cost.

Private insurance refers to coverage people can buy from private companies to help fund the costs of health care services.

In **two-tier health systems** the government provides basic health services at no cost to the user, but a second tier of faster and higher-quality services is available to people who can afford to pay for them.

◄ A government-run street hospital in Shenzhen, China, offers free or **subsidized** health care treatment for local residents. Services at the hospital include heath checks and skin-care treatment.

Learning about a new topic can be overwhelming. So, where do you begin? The Internet is a good source of information. For a global perspective on health care you might visit websites for **non-governmental organizations (NGOs)** such as the World Bank, United Nations (UN), and WHO. Look at each government's website for its own health care system, such as the U.S. Department of Health and Human Services or Health Canada. To get the most from your Internet research, do a targeted search using specific keywords related to universal health care. Use a variety of search engines, such as Google, Yahoo!, and Bing, as each one may produce slightly different results.

LIBRARIES AND THINK TANKS

Libraries are another great place to build background knowledge. They contain books, magazines, journals, newspapers, and other information you might not be able to find using an Internet search. Hospital and medical libraries provide a wealth of information related to the health field, including information on policies, research, and regulatory activities. Librarians can help you quickly find information on your subject.

Other places to look for background information include **think tanks** dedicated to the health care industry. They may have reports or offer ideas and advice about the subject. The Alliance for Health Policy in the United States, the Institute of Health Economics in Canada, and the Health Foundation in the United Kingdom are think tanks that focus on health care.

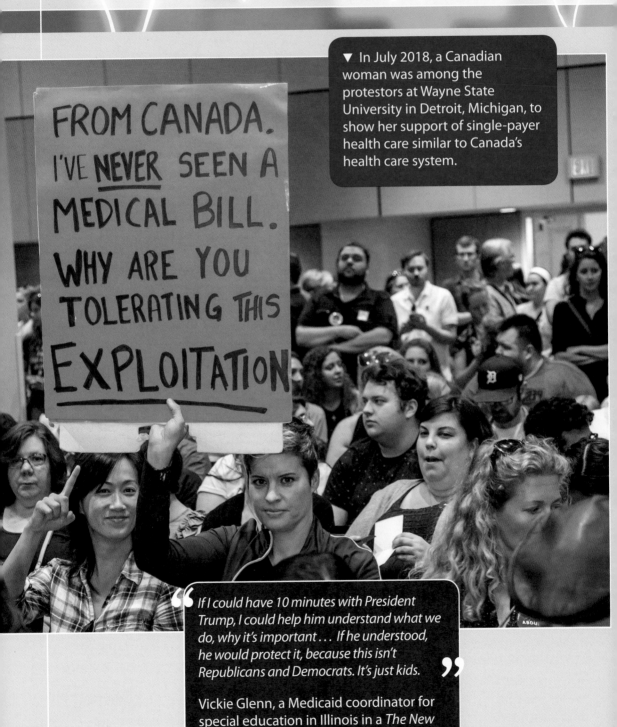

FROM CANADA.
I'VE NEVER SEEN A
MEDICAL BILL.
WHY ARE YOU
TOLERATING THIS
EXPLOITATION

▼ In July 2018, a Canadian woman was among the protestors at Wayne State University in Detroit, Michigan, to show her support of single-payer health care similar to Canada's health care system.

" If I could have 10 minutes with President Trump, I could help him understand what we do, why it's important … If he understood, he would protect it, because this isn't Republicans and Democrats. It's just kids. "

Vickie Glenn, a Medicaid coordinator for special education in Illinois in a *The New York Times* story, May 2017

Items that provide information about a subject are known as **source materials**. They can include documents, photographs, paintings, artifacts, **transcripts**, documentaries, books, and more. There are three main types of source materials: primary, secondary, and tertiary.

PRIMARY SOURCES

These are created by people with personal knowledge or experience of an event, situation, or location. They provide original first-hand accounts. Eyewitness reports, **statistical** data, recordings, original research, diaries, speeches, and emails are all examples.

Primary sources on universal health care include:
- government white papers, or reports, on health care funding models
- live television interviews with politicians and hospital representatives
- brochures outlining the services offered by health care providers
- rate cards for insurance companies
- images of protestors at a rally against health care cuts
- results from a phone survey on public satisfaction with local health care coverage
- blogs created by health care workers and **lobbyists**
- handwritten doctors' notes and **prescriptions**
- patient invoices for health care services.

SECONDARY AND TERTIARY SOURCES

Secondary sources are made by compiling, **analyzing**, and interpreting information found in primary sources. The information is modified, reorganized, and arranged in a new way. Secondary sources include newspaper stories written after an event takes place, biographies, movies, and **reference** books. Graphs, charts, and diagrams that represent statistical information visually are also examples.

Tertiary sources act as a reference tool to help you find more information about a subject. They include textbooks, dictionaries, encyclopedias, indexes, almanacs, and **bibliographies**.

▼ As a nation's population ages, so does its health care spending. Care for the elderly is one of the biggest burdens on health care systems. In the United States, the number of people more than age 65 is expected to double from about 50 million to 100 million by 2060.

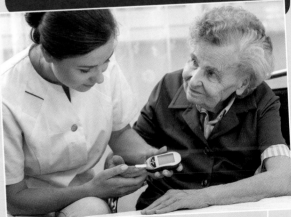

To interpret information is to make sense of it. However, not all information is easy to understand. Information that contains a lot of numbers and statistics can be difficult to make sense of. Often graphs and charts are used to organize data in a new way. It is easier to draw conclusions using visual aids. For instance, tables filled with numbers comparing how much money governments around the world spend on health care per person can be overwhelming. However, when shown as a bar chart (see page 7), they are much easier to interpret.

Before you delve into a topic, it is also important to find out if there are any key words or concepts that will help you make sense of the subject you are studying. Understanding the difference between private health coverage, Medicare, and tiered systems, for example, can help guide your research on universal health care.

▼ In February 2017, doctors were among protesters in Philadelphia, U.S.A., against changes to the Affordable Care Act (ACA). The ACA is a law that helps lower the costs of health care services so more people can afford them (see page 22 for more).

ASK YOUR OWN QUESTIONS

For each of your source materials, check: Has the author left out any facts or important information? Is the author trying to persuade you to feel a certain way? Does the author use extreme language? If **bias** is strong, you might not want to use the source.

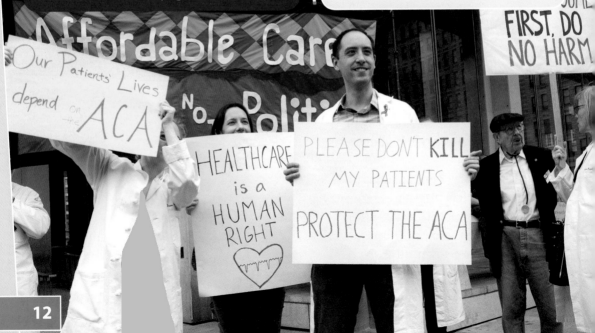

MEDICARE   **HEALTH INSURANCE**

1-800-MEDICARE (1-800-633-4227)

NAME OF BENEFICIARY
LARRY SUTTON

MEDICARE CLAIM NUMBER   SEX
925-42-9374-N   MALE

IS ENTITLED TO   EFFECTIVE DATE
HOSPITAL (PART A)   08-01-2015
MEDICAL (PART B)   08-01-2015

SIGN HERE ➡

▲ In the United States, Medicare includes hospital stays, care in a skilled nursing facility, hospice services, and home health care (Part A), as well as doctor visits, outpatient care, medical supplies, and preventive services (Part B).

EVALUATING A SOURCE

Some source materials will be more useful, valid, and relevant to your research than others. One way to tell if a source of information is high quality is to determine if it is **credible** and reliable. Source materials created by people with great experience, expertise, or **credentials** related to the topic tend to have more value. A top-quality source will contain quotations, a bibliography, and other evidence to support any facts or information presented. In addition, the information should be well organized and free of any grammatical or spelling errors.

Bias plays a big role in the credibility of source materials. Almost all sources of information contain some bias because every person or group in the world has its own opinions and perspectives on a topic. Unbiased source materials present a balanced view of the subject that is based on fact, not on opinion.

Sometimes creators of source materials unintentionally—or intentionally—include bias in their work. For instance, politicians who oppose universal health care may use language in their speeches that aims to persuade people to take their point of view. Similarly, a blogger with a large online audience who supports the concept of health care for everyone may try to gain support for the cause through social **media**. It is important to use a variety of source materials to ensure you have a balanced view of how universal health care impacts society. It will help you become a more informed citizen.

3

THE BIG PICTURE

For countries to grow and thrive socially and **economically**, their people need to be healthy and able to contribute to society. However, about 50 percent of people across the world do not have access to essential health services, such as **prenatal** care, child **immunization**, and access to clean water and sanitation. More than 800 million people globally spend 10 percent or more of their total household budget to pay for health care. A further 100 million or so people have been pushed into extreme **poverty** because they have to pay their own health care expenses.

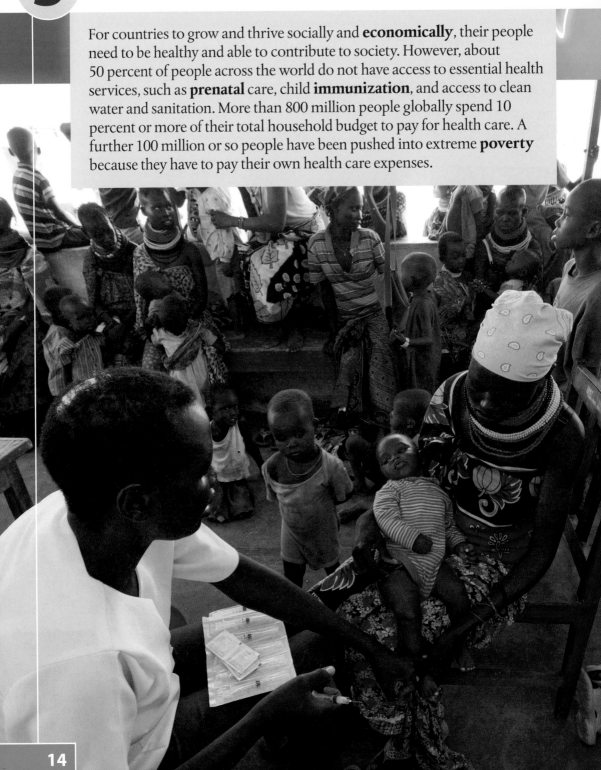

THE CENTRAL ISSUES

What are the risks countries face by not putting a universal health care system in place? Are there any alternatives to universal health care that could provide support at a lower cost to the public?

Typically, countries with universal health care programs provide coverage for everyone from birth to death. This has an important impact on the health of society as a whole. Early access to health care helps children get off to a healthy start in life. Studies show that healthy children grow into healthy adults. One reason is because preventive care is a big part of universal health care. It means children receive treatments such as vaccines that help to prevent diseases. They also get regular checkups to identify potential health issues in their early, more treatable, stages.

Education programs that teach children how to take better care of themselves and make healthier choices, such as eating a balanced diet, also play a major role in universal health care systems. As adults, these citizens put less stress on the health system because they often require minimal care.

COST ISSUES

Universal health care helps ensure people have better physical and mental health overall. This is good for everyone in a society. Free or cheap health services help support a nation's economy so it can continue to grow and develop. One reason for this is because universal health care reduces the risk of poverty for people who must borrow money to pay for health services. Another reason is that universal heath care increases the chance of people detecting illnesses early. As a result, they can get proper treatment, which costs less than ongoing care, and it leads to less sick time off education and work.

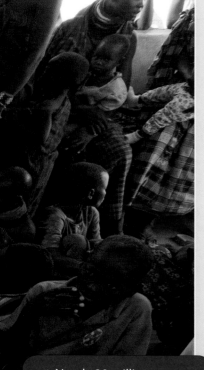

◄ Nearly 20 million children across the globe do not have access to life-saving vaccines. World Vision is one of the many nonprofit groups that provide vaccinations to children in need in countries such as Kenya.

Providing health coverage for all citizens of a country is not a new concept. It is rooted in the idea of **social welfare**, or social services and income security programs such as old age pensions, child benefits, or support for the unemployed or disabled. Most social welfare programs are put in place to overcome a social problem such as poverty or unemployment.

One of the earliest examples of a social welfare program dates back to 1601, when England's Queen Elizabeth I created the Act for Relief of the Poor. At the time in England, there were many poor people begging on the streets. The law was an effort to punish and prevent begging and deal with a failing economy. It gave the English government the right to collect taxes from property owners to provide assistance for the poor, disabled, elderly, and sick who could not work. The Poor Law remained in effect for more than 230 years.

MODERN WELFARE SYSTEMS

Modern social welfare systems first appeared in Germany in the late 1800s. A new political party had formed in Germany. It promoted better rights for the working class and **socialist** ideals that the government did not want to grow in popularity. To make party supporters happy, the country brought in several social welfare programs. These included pensions, accident insurance, and a system of health coverage.

France and other European nations soon set up similar systems based on this German model. The United Kingdom created its National Insurance Act in 1911. It provided both health and unemployment insurance benefits for industrial workers.

KEY PLAYERS

Florence Nightingale was a British nurse in the mid-1800s. At that time, hospitals in Britain were crowded, dirty, and in bad shape, especially those found in workhouses that were part of the Poor Law reforms. Diseases and infections spread quickly through these hospitals. Nightingale called on the British government to raise the quality of health care for everyone, including the poor. Nightingale developed hospital design standards and practices to improve care, safety, and cleanliness.

Countries all over the world looked to her for advice. Nightingale also created training programs for nurses and set high standards for nursing that helped make it a respected profession.

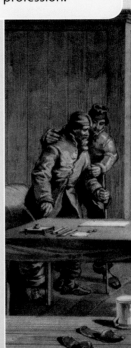

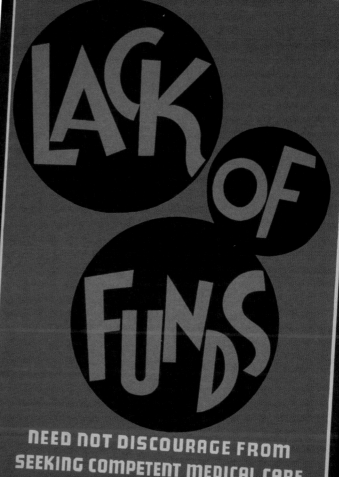

▶ This poster from the 1930s helped promote better health care in the United States. It was created at a time when many people were out of work and without money to pay for health care.

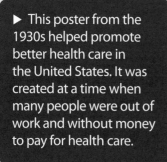

▼ British soldiers injured during the Crimean War were sent across the Black Sea to military hospitals, such as this one in Scutari (now called Üsküdar) in Istanbul, Turkey, where Florence Nightingale worked.

LACK OF FUNDS

NEED NOT DISCOURAGE FROM SEEKING COMPETENT MEDICAL CARE

consult your health bureau

WPA FEDERAL ART PROJECT   DIS. ½

Countries put health care programs in place for a variety of reasons. For instance, in Russia in 1917 the citizens threatened to stop supporting the government if it did not provide social welfare systems that included affordable health care. A group known as the **Bolsheviks** overthrew the government in what is known as the October **Revolution**. The revolution led to changes in the Russian economy that included the creation of a free health care system and other social welfare programs.

In countries such as Belgium and Spain, health care programs solved a problem in the workplace. Often, workers were taking too much time off work due to illness. The nation's economies received a boost by

THE NEW
NATIONAL
HEALTH
SERVICE

*

Your new National Health Service begins on 5th July. What is it? How do you get it?

It will provide you with all medical, dental, and nursing care. Everyone—rich or poor, man, woman or child—can use it or any part of it. There are no charges, except for a few special items. There are no insurance qualifications. But it is not a "charity". You are all paying for it, mainly as taxpayers, and it will relieve your money worries in time of illness.

▲ Britain's National Health Service (NHS), set up in 1948, is tax-funded and aims to provide health care for all with no out-of-pocket costs for users.

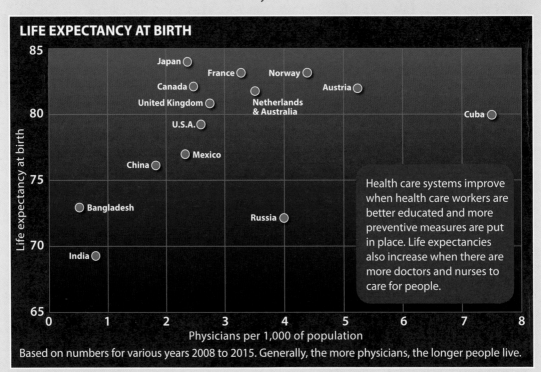

LIFE EXPECTANCY AT BIRTH

Life expectancy at birth

Japan, France, Canada, Norway, Austria, United Kingdom, Netherlands & Australia, Cuba, U.S.A., Mexico, China, Bangladesh, Russia, India

Physicians per 1,000 of population

Health care systems improve when health care workers are better educated and more preventive measures are put in place. Life expectancies also increase when there are more doctors and nurses to care for people.

Based on numbers for various years 2008 to 2015. Generally, the more physicians, the longer people live.

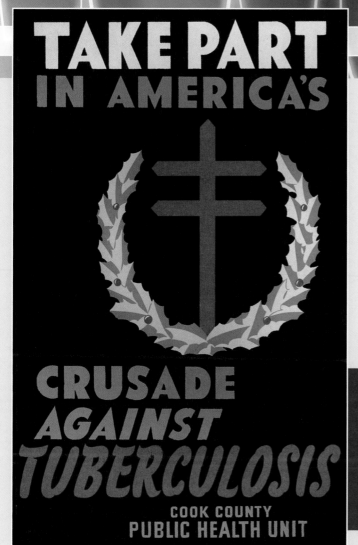

TAKE PART IN AMERICA'S CRUSADE AGAINST TUBERCULOSIS

COOK COUNTY
PUBLIC HEALTH UNIT

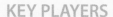

KEY PLAYERS

The **World Health Organization (WHO)** is a specialized agency of the United Nations. It is made up of 193 member states from every continent who all support the goal of better health for everyone in all parts of the world. WHO was founded in Geneva, Switzerland, on April 7, 1948. April 7 is now celebrated as World Health Day each year.

◀ In the 1940s, tuberculosis (TB) cases were rising in Chicago, Illinois. This poster was part of an education **campaign** by the government to encourage people to get tested for the highly **contagious** disease to help prevent its spread.

having healthy workers who took fewer sick days. Ireland's health care program prevented the spread of contagious diseases, such as tuberculosis, which killed thousands of people. Making sure everyone had access to vaccines and other preventive measures helped solve the issue.

By the 1930s, most countries in Western and Central Europe had established some form of nationwide health program to increase their productivity. Japan, Australia, and New Zealand had formed their own health insurance systems or free public hospital care for people in need. Following World War II (1939–1945), other countries began to bring in a universal health care system. Some chose to expand existing health care systems, while others built entirely new systems. Northern European countries also created their own universal health care systems in the 1950s and 1960s.

In Canada's early history, people paid doctors and hospitals directly for their services. People who could not pay did not receive care. Most doctors adjusted their rates based on how much a patient could afford. The wealthy usually paid higher fees than the poor. When the **Great Depression** began in 1929, only about 40 percent of Canadians could afford to pay for health care. Up to one quarter of the population was unemployed and hungry.

The Depression and the effect it had on people slowly led to the creation of a system of social welfare programs funded and delivered through tax dollars. These included "relief" to help people left destitute. As the economy suffered, everyone struggled to pay their bills. Hospitals closed. Over the next two decades, attempts were made at the provincial and national levels to expand

ASK YOUR OWN QUESTIONS

Why do you think health care was such an important issue during the Great Depression? How did the Canadian government finally secure the money to fund a health care program? Why might doctors and the federal government have opposed the program at first?

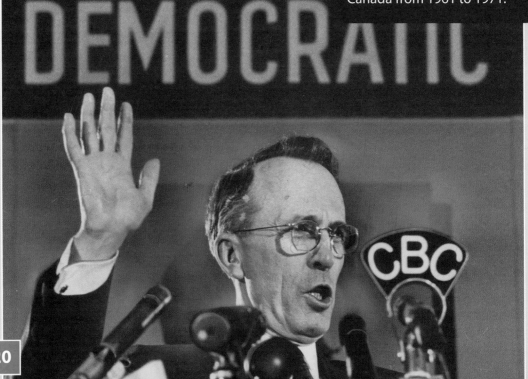

▼ Tommy Douglas was Leader of the New Democratic Party in Canada from 1961 to 1971.

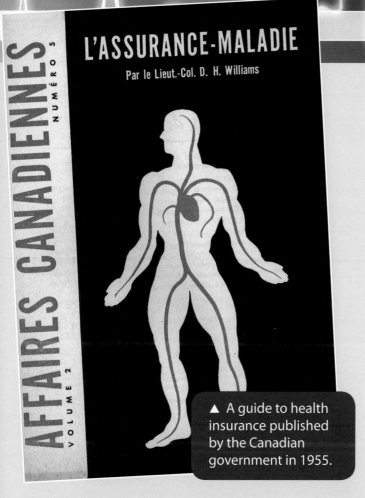

L'ASSURANCE-MALADIE

Par le Lieut.-Col. D. H. Williams

AFFAIRES CANADIENNES

NUMÉRO 5

VOLUME 2

▲ A guide to health insurance published by the Canadian government in 1955.

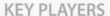

KEY PLAYERS

Tommy Douglas was a minister who lived in Weyburn, Saskatchewan. He saw first-hand how the Great Depression and drought had impacted farmers in Saskatchewan. They had no money for food, schools, or health care. He set up classes in his church and held food drives, but he felt the government could do more to help. He eventually became involved in politics and was elected premier of Saskatchewan in 1944. He immediately began establishing policies to help farmers in need. Douglas is known as the father of Medicare in Canada.

social welfare to include health care. None of the plans were introduced.

COST ISSUES

Medicare, the government-funded universal health insurance program, began as a provincial program in Saskatchewan in 1962. It was the first government-controlled universal medical insurance plan in North America. Saskatchewan premier Tommy Douglas proposed it much earlier, but funding was not available. Then, in 1957, the federal government passed a law to provide funding for 50 percent of hospital expenses for provincial and territorial governments. As a result, Saskatchewan moved ahead with its public health plan in 1962. Other provinces soon followed. In 1966, Prime Minister Lester B. Pearson brought in the Medical Care Act, which extended health insurance to cover doctors' services. The Canada Health Act, passed in 1984, ended user fees and direct billing by doctors. Today, the publicly funded, single-payer health care system remains a key part of the Canadian social welfare system. Proponents now want to improve and expand it.

Prior to World War I (1914–1918), the U.S. government made several attempts to move toward a national health system. However, every attempt was met with objection from doctors, businesses, insurance companies, and others. Still, the nation successfully adopted other social welfare programs. President Franklin Delano Roosevelt signed the Social Security Act into effect in 1935 at the height of the Great Depression. The act helped create economic security for all U.S. citizens through an **income tax**. Over time and despite initial opposition, the act became an important aspect of social welfare in the United States.

Attempts to create a universal health care system have not been met with the same enthusiasm in the United States. During World War II, there was a labor shortage as men went off to fight. Workers were in high demand, and companies were willing to pay to hold on to them. President Roosevelt froze wages to prevent them from skyrocketing due to the demand. Companies looked for other ways to entice workers such as health coverage. After the war, companies were given tax breaks to continue to pay for employee health care. A massive private health industry developed as a result.

MEDICARE AND MEDICAID
Over the next several decades, different health care plans were proposed by presidents Harry S. Truman, John F. Kennedy, and others, but the American Medical Association (AMA) fought against them, as doctors would lose part of their income and their **autonomy**.

In 1965, President Lyndon B. Johnson created two social welfare programs: Medicare for people more than age 65 and Medicaid for people with a low income. The Affordable Care Act of 2010 required all U.S. citizens to purchase health insurance as a way to lower health care costs overall. Some people would have to pay for health care services even if they did not use them to offset the cost of caring for the sick and elderly who use the services more often.

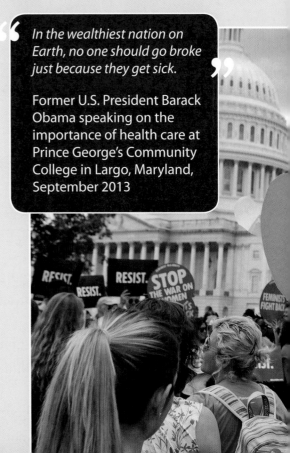

> *In the wealthiest nation on Earth, no one should go broke just because they get sick.*

Former U.S. President Barack Obama speaking on the importance of health care at Prince George's Community College in Largo, Maryland, September 2013

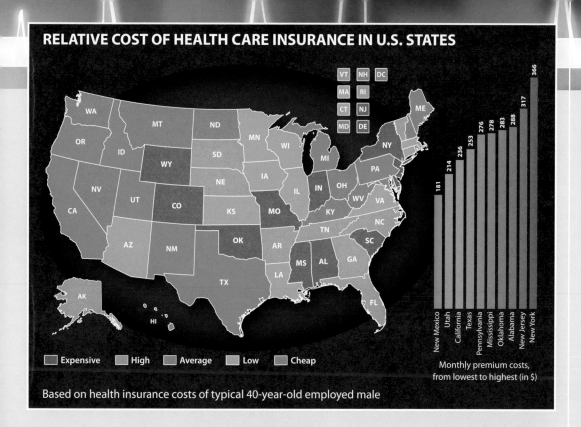

RELATIVE COST OF HEALTH CARE INSURANCE IN U.S. STATES

Expensive · High · Average · Low · Cheap

Based on health insurance costs of typical 40-year-old employed male

Monthly premium costs, from lowest to highest (in $)

New Mexico	181
Utah	214
California	236
Texas	253
Pennsylvania	276
Mississippi	278
Oklahoma	283
Alabama	288
New Jersey	317
New York	366

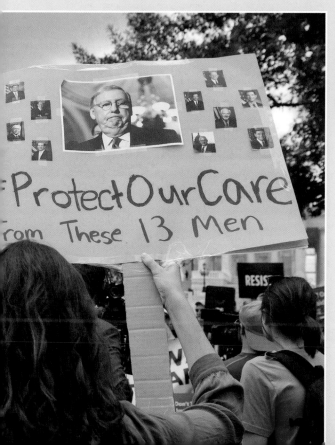

◄ On June 27, 2017, protestors gathered outside the U.S. Capitol building to voice their disapproval of cuts to the Affordable Care Act.

THE CENTRAL ISSUES

What shortfalls does social security in the United States face today? How does this help reinforce the idea that a nationwide public health program would be a burden on the country?

There are many different perspectives—both positive and negative—on the issue of health care for all. Federal and local governments, international organizations, insurance companies, employers, hospitals, long-term care facilities, and the general public all have their own views on the subject. It is important to consider a variety of perspectives to help balance your own view. Seeing an issue through someone else's eyes can change the way you see it and shape your conclusions.

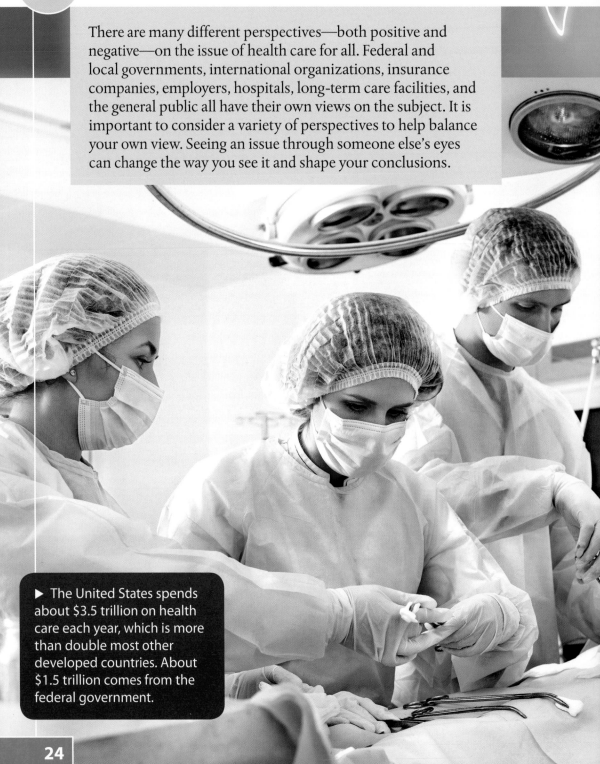

▶ The United States spends about $3.5 trillion on health care each year, which is more than double most other developed countries. About $1.5 trillion comes from the federal government.

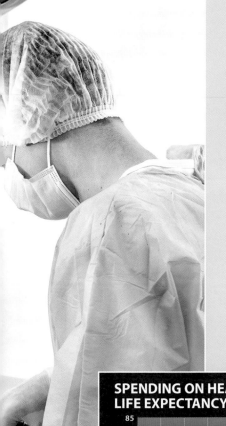

INFORMATION LITERACY

Being able to quickly and easily locate relevant and reliable source materials is an important part of getting and staying informed. Information literacy involves sorting, understanding, and analyzing your materials and deciding which of them are the most important and why. When you have strong information literacy skills, you can evaluate information critically and competently.

Keep in mind that not everything you read is true, especially on the Internet. There are nearly two billion websites and many are owned by individuals whose information is not vetted for accuracy. Anyone can post anything on their personal websites, whether or not the information is true. Free speech laws prevent **censorship** in many parts of the world. Health care lobbyists use websites to promote their cause. Doctors may use the Internet to sell their services. Governments often post information about preventive care and treatment.

It is important to evaluate every source based on its relevance, authority, and accuracy. Governments, nonprofit organizations, education institutes, and well-known news agencies are all a good place to look for trusted information.

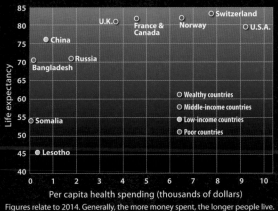

SPENDING ON HEALTH CARE RELATED TO LIFE EXPECTANCY

Life expectancy (vertical axis, 40 to 85)
Per capita health spending (thousands of dollars) (horizontal axis, 0 to 10)

Data points:
- U.K.
- France & Canada
- Norway
- Switzerland
- U.S.A.
- China
- Russia
- Bangladesh
- Somalia
- Lesotho

Legend:
- Wealthy countries
- Middle-income countries
- Low-income countries
- Poor countries

Figures relate to 2014. Generally, the more money spent, the longer people live.

▶ The 2007 documentary *Sicko* by filmmaker Michael Moore explores why so many U.S. citizens do not have health coverage and how it has impacted their lives.

▼ In Canada, depending on the province, government grants cover from 70 to 100 percent of running costs for hospitals. Many hospitals, such as the Alberta Children's Hospital, hold fundraisers, accept charitable donations, charge for parking, or sell items in a gift shop to supplement any remaining costs.

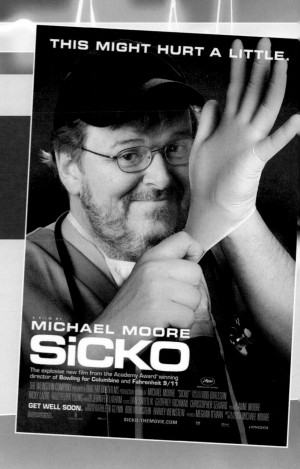

THIS MIGHT HURT A LITTLE.

A FILM BY
MICHAEL MOORE
SiCKO

The explosive new film from the Academy Award® winning director of **Bowling for Columbine** and **Fahrenheit 9/11**

GET WELL SOON.

SICKO-THEMOVIE.COM

LIONSGATE

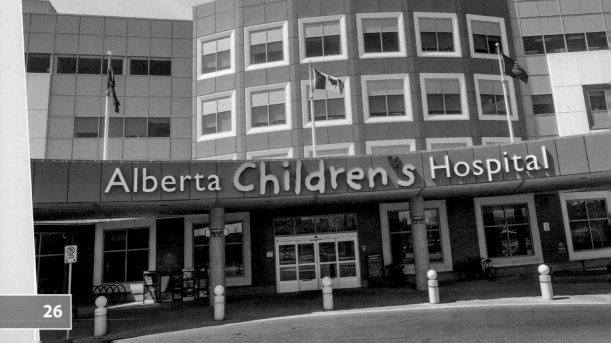

Alberta Children's Hospital

Governments must juggle health care budgets wisely and often take money from other services, such as transportation and education, to fund them. As a result, most universal health care programs cover only basic services at no personal direct cost at the time of use. Of the 32 developed nations that have universal health care programs, most employ one of three common models.

THREE DIFFERENT SYSTEMS

First, in single-payer systems, the government charges income taxes, which are used to help pay for health care. While tax-funded health care is a huge expenditure, the government controls charges for it, so costs are lower than privately funded systems.

In the United Kingdom, for example, tax-funded government programs cover about 85 percent of health care spending. Private insurance covers the remaining 15 percent of health care expenses. Canada uses a similar scheme. About 70 percent of health care expenses are paid for through money from federal, provincial, territorial, and local governments, plus other social security plans. The rest is paid for by the patient or private funding sources such as insurance companies. These cover the cost of medications outside a hospital setting, eyeglasses, and dental care. Doctors are not government employees. Most are paid on a fee-for-service basis

—creating concerns for some patients about the quality of their services.

Second, some countries have a **mandatory** health insurance system. In Germany, for example, people who earn less than a certain amount each year must buy into the government health insurance program. The funds are pooled with government tax money to provide care for everyone in Germany. There is also a private health insurance program that higher-income people can choose to opt into as well.

Third, in countries where there is a two-tier health care system, such as in France and Australia, the government pays for basic health care services through taxes. A second tier of health care that provides faster and better quality services is available for those who can afford to pay for it.

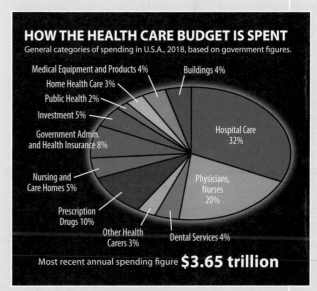

HOW THE HEALTH CARE BUDGET IS SPENT
General categories of spending in U.S.A., 2018, based on government figures.

Medical Equipment and Products 4%
Home Health Care 3%
Public Health 2%
Investment 5%
Government Admin. and Health Insurance 8%
Nursing and Care Homes 5%
Prescription Drugs 10%
Other Health Carers 3%
Dental Services 4%
Buildings 4%
Hospital Care 32%
Physicians, Nurses 20%

Most recent annual spending figure **$3.65 trillion**

In many parts of the world, there are not enough qualified medical professionals to provide the required health care services. Since universal health care programs provide equal access for all, they put greater stress on doctors who are already overburdened. Often, there are not enough doctors to help everyone. Still, medical professionals are typically in favor of these programs. Most doctors do not want to turn away people who need their help but cannot afford it.

Universal health care also covers public health measures for entire populations such as immunization programs and controlling mosquitoes in infested areas. The result of these measures is a healthier overall population. This leads to better performance at work as a healthy workforce means fewer people take time off in sick days or wait an illness out until they are so sick they have to visit a hospital emergency room.

THE INSURANCE FACTOR

More than half of all U.S. doctors support universal health care programs because they provide consistent coverage for patients. Doctors also face less hassle than working with insurance companies that want to save money rather than lives. **Administrative** costs are lower since there are standardized ways of doing things and service providers need only to deal directly with the government rather than various insurance providers.

Yet there are some drawbacks to the single-payer method that medical professionals would rather limit by allowing some private insurance options to remain intact. This is largely due to the fact that private insurers pay doctors and hospitals at higher rates than Medicare.

ASK YOUR OWN QUESTIONS

Do you think people would be more likely to visit the doctor, even when they do not really need to, if they do not have to pay directly out of pocket for the visit? Do the benefits of universal health care outweigh the risks?

"
Obviously, education is hugely important, along with health care. They're the basics and you're hurting your own country if you don't pour money into them. "

British actress Kelly Reilly expressed her thoughts on health care during an interview with *The Guardian*, 2011

▶ Mobile health clinics, such as the Pathway to Health in California, bring medical, surgical, dental, eyecare, and other services to different communities. Often, they provide their services free of charge to people in need such as those who do not have health insurance coverage.

28

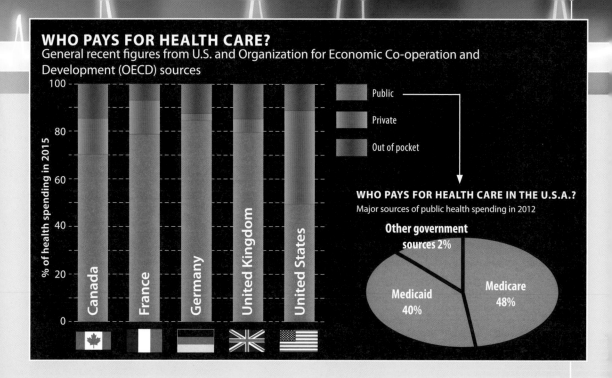

WHO PAYS FOR HEALTH CARE?

General recent figures from U.S. and Organization for Economic Co-operation and Development (OECD) sources

% of health spending in 2015

- Public
- Private
- Out of pocket

Canada
France
Germany
United Kingdom
United States

WHO PAYS FOR HEALTH CARE IN THE U.S.A.?

Major sources of public health spending in 2012

Other government sources 2%

Medicaid 40%

Medicare 48%

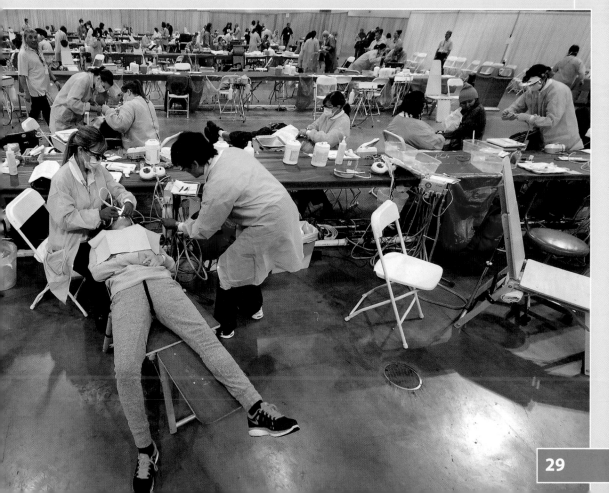

Private insurance provides people who can afford it the opportunity to buy medical services from non-government suppliers. This may give them access to better quality and faster services, and to expensive prescription drugs. Private insurance is voluntary—people can choose to buy it. Universal health care programs are mandatory.

According to WHO, France's two-tier health care system is one of the best in the world. In this system, since there are both **regulated** public service providers and unregulated private providers, health care costs vary. The government covers about 80 percent of the anticipated cost of treatment, not what the patient actually pays. Many people purchase private insurance to help cover the extra costs.

THE HIGH COST OF PREMIUMS

In the United States, unless you qualify for a social welfare program such as Medicare or Medicaid, the only way to get health care services is to pay out of pocket, purchase private insurance, or take a job that provides insurance as a benefit.

A risk is that many insurance companies charge high premiums for certain conditions or will not cover them at all. For many U.S. citizens, their top concern is accessing affordable health care, with some turning to **crowdfunding** and other means to help cover mounting debt from paying for costly health services such as cancer treatments. For instance, the cost of giving birth in a U.S. hospital is more than $30,000, leaving uninsured mothers with huge bills if they do not qualify for Medicaid. Before calling an ambulance, many people must first consider if their insurance will cover it because they cannot afford to pay out of pocket for the service.

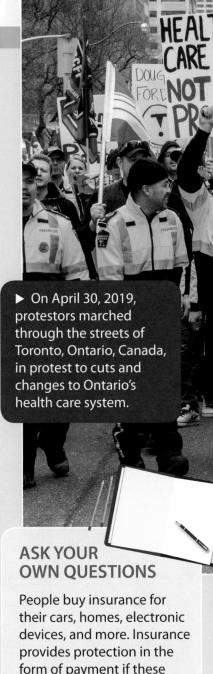

▶ On April 30, 2019, protestors marched through the streets of Toronto, Ontario, Canada, in protest to cuts and changes to Ontario's health care system.

ASK YOUR OWN QUESTIONS

People buy insurance for their cars, homes, electronic devices, and more. Insurance provides protection in the form of payment if these items are damaged or lost. Does this make health care insurance acceptable? Why or why not?

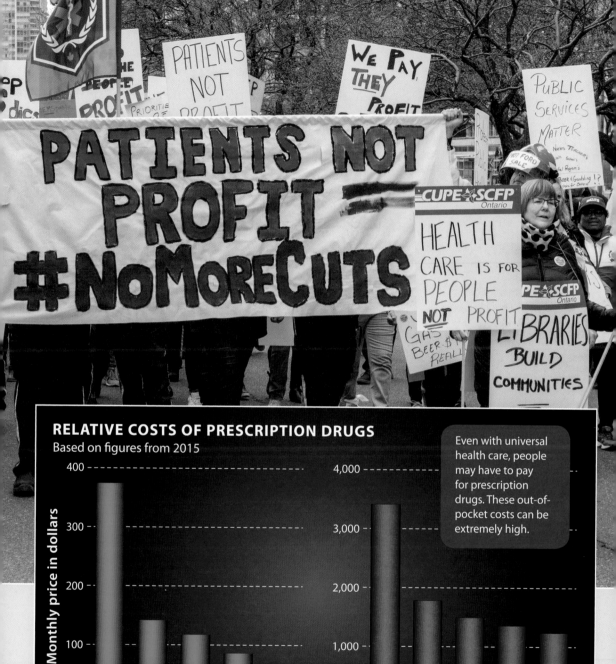

RELATIVE COSTS OF PRESCRIPTION DRUGS

Based on figures from 2015

Even with universal health care, people may have to pay for prescription drugs. These out-of-pocket costs can be extremely high.

Monthly price in dollars

Lantus
(long-acting insulin)

U.S.A. — China — Saudi Arabia — Brazil — Canada

Humira
(rheumatoid arthritis self-injection)

U.S.A. — Germany — Brazil — Saudi Arabia — Australia

Employers often help pay for health care coverage or private insurance as an added-bonus, or benefit, for working with them. Providing health care benefits leads to a more productive workforce as employees are less likely to become sick and have better emotional well-being. In the United States, people must pay for their own health insurance, so many employers offer to pay for basic medical coverage as a way to encourage the person to take a job with their company. Many U.S. citizens take jobs specifically for the health benefits.

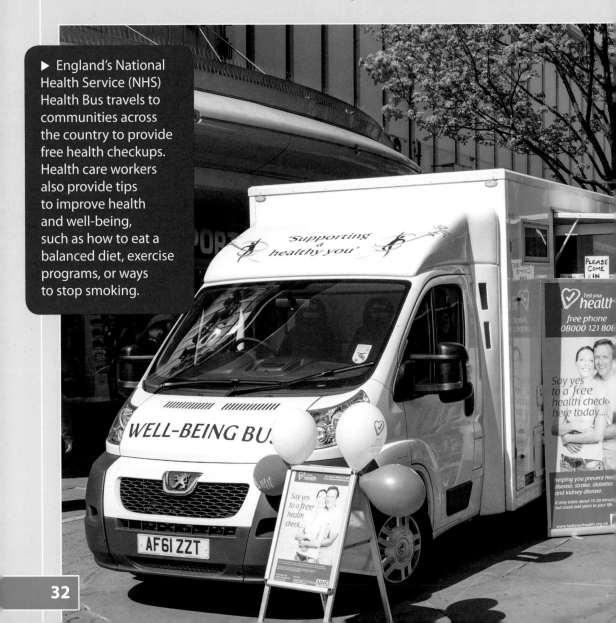

▶ England's National Health Service (NHS) Health Bus travels to communities across the country to provide free health checkups. Health care workers also provide tips to improve health and well-being, such as how to eat a balanced diet, exercise programs, or ways to stop smoking.

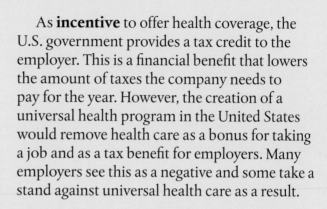

WHAT'S AT STAKE?

Health insurance programs cost companies thousands of dollars per employee, so why would they want to offer them? Should employees have the option to opt out of health care programs if their partner already pays into one or if they do not want to share costs?

As **incentive** to offer health coverage, the U.S. government provides a tax credit to the employer. This is a financial benefit that lowers the amount of taxes the company needs to pay for the year. However, the creation of a universal health program in the United States would remove health care as a bonus for taking a job and as a tax benefit for employers. Many employers see this as a negative and some take a stand against universal health care as a result.

EMPLOYER-SPONSORED SCHEMES

Universal health care systems often do not cover all health expenses. Employers may offer to help pay for private insurance benefits to cover additional services such as dental care, eyeglasses, and prescription drugs. In Canada, many employers, but not all, offer to pay for extra private health insurance, a savings of thousands of dollars per year per family.

While an employer-sponsored insurance program is a nice incentive, it is not the only factor to consider. Work schedules, location, parental leave, vacation days, and office culture are just as important in an employee's decision-making process. Some people may prefer to work from home or have a parking space near the office rather than health coverage.

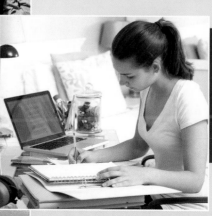

◄ Most employers put details of the health care insurance plan on their website for staff and jobseekers to review.

Most people living in developed countries accept that their government charges taxes to provide social welfare benefits. In the long run, universal health care costs less in taxpayers' dollars if the system works well. This is because healthy citizens are more active in their communities. They are better able to hold down jobs and are more productive because they take fewer sick days. In turn, they pay taxes and contribute to the social welfare system. Even in the United States, where there is strong opposition to universal health care, there is a great deal of government support for social welfare programs that benefit the greater good, including Medicaid and Medicare.

U.S. COSTS AND BENEFITS

The United States has the most expensive health care system in the world. On average, the country pays out more than $10,000 per person annually for health care, which is more than double the budget of other developed

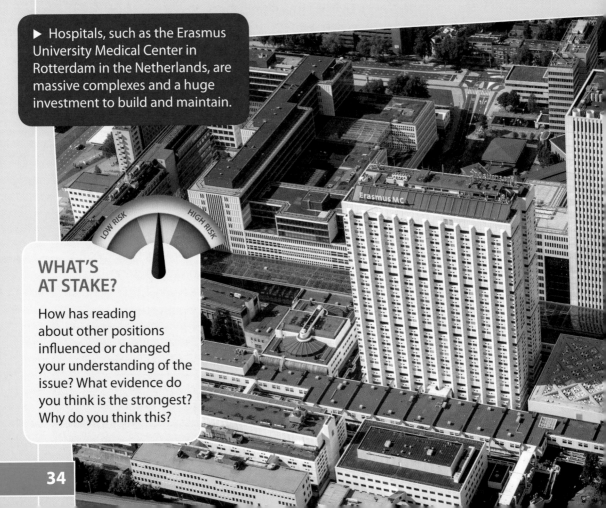

▶ Hospitals, such as the Erasmus University Medical Center in Rotterdam in the Netherlands, are massive complexes and a huge investment to build and maintain.

WHAT'S AT STAKE?

How has reading about other positions influenced or changed your understanding of the issue? What evidence do you think is the strongest? Why do you think this?

LOW RISK   HIGH RISK

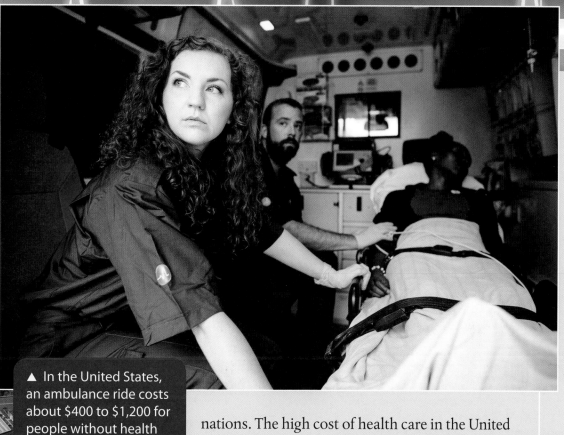

▲ In the United States, an ambulance ride costs about $400 to $1,200 for people without health insurance, depending on the locations and services provided.

nations. The high cost of health care in the United States is largely due to the high costs being charged for services by private health care providers. A **CT scan** in the United States costs nearly $900 compared to $279 in the Netherlands and only $97 in Canada. Similarly, wages are higher in the United States. Health care workers who specialize in a certain field earn well over $300,000 compared with $100,000 in Sweden and $200,000 in Australia. Yet, 28 percent of U.S. citizens have more than one chronic condition such as diabetes or heart disease—a higher rate than in many other countries.

There are many valuable benefits to the U.S. health system, however. U.S. citizens have fast and efficient access to health services including scans, specialists, cancer treatment, and more. They also have better access than others to new treatments for chronic diseases. U.S. hospitals are also more likely to invest in cutting-edge medical technologies and clinical studies.

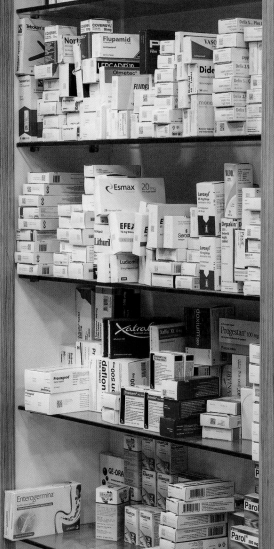
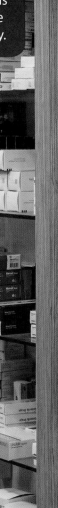

5 STAYING INFORMED

Once you get informed about a topic, it is just as important to stay informed. Information, including facts and points of view, change all the time. What was accurate or common practice in the past may not be today. Keeping current on the latest details helps you make appropriate decisions as an informed citizen.

▶ A feature of most universal health care programs is the low cost of prescription drugs so it is affordable for people to get the drugs they need to stay healthy.

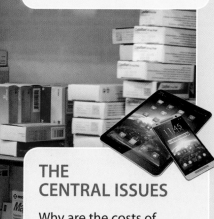

THE CENTRAL ISSUES

Why are the costs of prescription drugs so high in the United States (see page 31)? What can be done to lower these costs and ensure people get the medications they need?

In 2012, the UN endorsed a **resolution** on global health and foreign policy to urge member nations to take urgent steps to improve their health care systems and work toward the goal of implementing universal health programs. Three years later, all UN member states committed to do their best to create universal health care systems by 2030. It was part of the resolution on Transforming Our World: The 2030 Agenda for Sustainable Development.

Under this initiative, UN member countries must look for ways to provide access to quality essential services, such as medicines and vaccines for all, by 2030. They must also find ways to fund health care programs so that people do not have to go into debt to access the care they need.

INTERNATIONAL ACTION

On December 12, 2017, the UN passed a third resolution as part of the global health and foreign policy initiative. The goal of this resolution was to encourage member states to educate local citizens, groups, and organizations on the issue of health care and to encourage them to contribute to the international effort.

Later, the UN declared the date December 12 as International Universal Health Coverage Day. On this day each year, **advocates** for universal health care speak up on behalf of the millions who do not have access to quality health services. They share stories of people in need and what has been accomplished to date in terms of access to health services. They also urge world leaders to invest in health care for all by 2030.

One organization involved in the 2030 health initiative is the Joint Learning Network (JLN) for Universal Health Coverage. JLN is made up of health care experts who work with governments and health and finance agencies from 34 countries. Together, they look for issues that might prevent JLN member countries from putting universal health care systems in place.

JLN designed a method to show how well a country's health care programs are working. In 2014, four countries tested the method: India, Indonesia, Ghana, and Malaysia. JLN analyzed the results and gave each country ideas on how to improve health care. In India, JLN found it was difficult to attract health workers to remote areas and programs would have to aim at fixing that. In Ghana, JLN discovered a lack of funding for disease prevention programs. In Malaysia, the five companies that provide the majority of health care in the country did not know about national health policies and procedures.

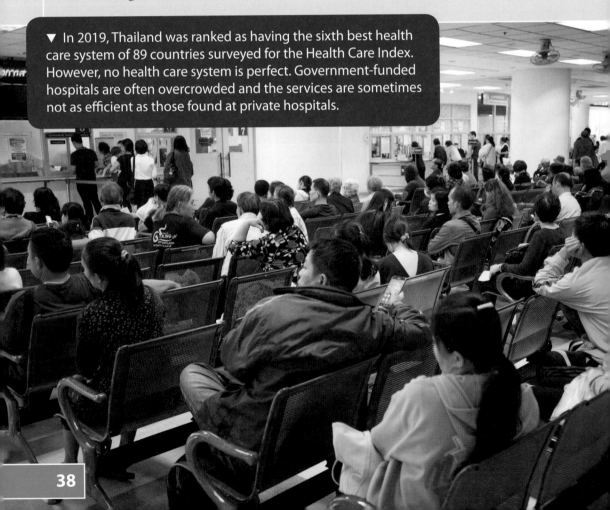

▼ In 2019, Thailand was ranked as having the sixth best health care system of 89 countries surveyed for the Health Care Index. However, no health care system is perfect. Government-funded hospitals are often overcrowded and the services are sometimes not as efficient as those found at private hospitals.

HELPING POOR COUNTRIES

Bangladesh is one of the poorest countries in the world. Its health care system relies on the government, private for-profit providers, charities, and international development agencies. As a result, 67 percent of people pay out of pocket for health care. To meet some of the UN's Sustainable Development Goals, Bangladesh relies on international development agencies such as Britain's UKAID. Under its Urban Health Systems Strengthening Project, UKAID has provided free basic health care to the extreme poor in that country. UKAID is also funding a program in Malawi, in Africa, that helps provide the tools and training health care workers need to ensure medicines reach patients.

> *America's health care system is neither healthy, caring, nor a system.*
> U.S. broadcast journalist Walter Cronkite, 1990

▼ Awareness campaigns to help educate and prevent the spread of contagious diseases are an important part of universal health care programs. The goal is to prevent disease before it occurs. In poorer countries without universal health care, aid agencies may provide basic care and assistance.

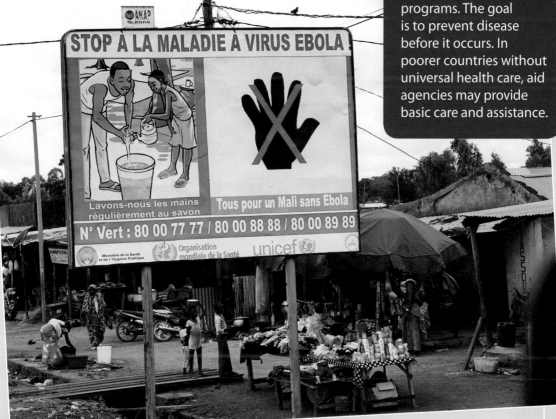

PLAN OF ACTION

By now, you have a good understanding of what universal health care is and how it started. New information is always coming to the forefront. Health care policies, practices, and funding models are constantly changing. Governments may decide a different health system is better for their country or that they need to focus their attention on other issues such as education. What was true one day may not be the next day. For this reason, it is important to stay up to date on current affairs.

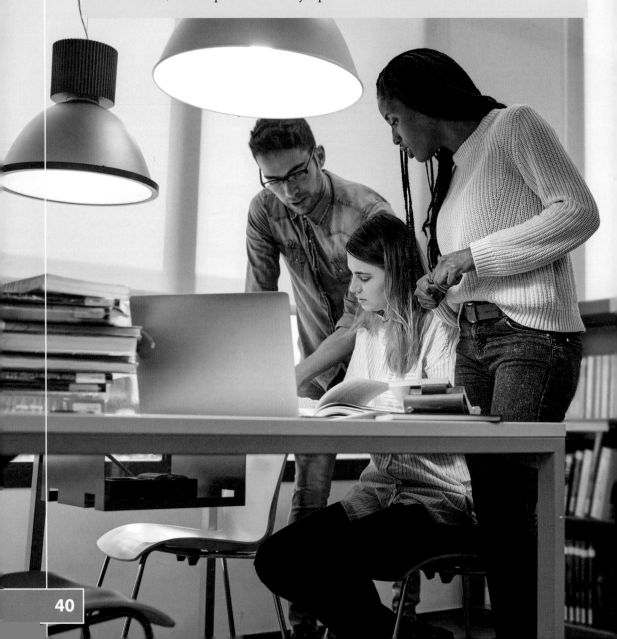

◄ When researching a topic, such as universal health care, share your thoughts, ideas, and opinions with other students, teachers, and your family.

INFORMATION EVERYWHERE
One of the best things about the Internet is having information available when it is convenient for you to access it. Unlike TV or radio programs that require you to tune in at a specific time, you can access information online from any place and at any time. In addition, you can find information from all over the world, giving you a global perspective. Local media may focus mainly on events that are important in your community or country, so you may not get the full picture.

There is no limit to the information you can access online, so branch out and look for information sources in other parts of the world. Gaining insight from international sources helps broaden and balance your perspective.

MEDIA LITERACY
Keep in mind that the media sometimes crafts messages in a way that can influence what you think, feel, and believe. Be aware of bias, and pay attention to the facts. Check information against a variety of sources to verify its accuracy. Most importantly, do not believe all you read or see.

Create a news diet of trustworthy sources to help you stay informed. To begin with, set up Google Alerts on universal health care to send the latest online posts to your email. You can also tune into respected news and radio shows or listen to podcasts that feature health care experts. Other great ways to stay current on health care is to read journal articles or to follow advocates and leaders on social media.

Currently, 58 countries have universal health care programs in place. Many humanitarian aid organizations and NGOs operate under the belief that everyone deserves the right to equal, affordable health care regardless of their race, gender, income, and other factors. Quality, accessible health care programs create a healthier, more productive population and reduce the risk of poverty for people who cannot afford to pay for health services. Yet despite the efforts of many countries, achieving the goal of quality health care for all is still a long way off for many nations.

Even for developed nations, health care is often a struggle to achieve and maintain. To establish universal health care, countries need to first set up a stable government framework in which to operate and provide the system. Also, to meet the 2030 target, more than 40 million more health care workers are needed worldwide, particularly in low- and lower-middle income countries. In the United States, politicians continue to debate the best and most **equitable** universal health care options to meet the needs of its citizens.

GETTING INVOLVED

Now that you are informed about universal health care, how do you feel about it? Do you think having a quality public health care system provides value to a country or is it a draw on funds that could be used elsewhere? What can you do to show your support for or against it? You might choose to join a rally, write to a local politician, or create a website that expresses your perspective on health care. Whether or not you choose to take action, getting informed and staying informed is a good first step toward becoming an involved citizen and forming a balanced view of the issue.

SEARCH TIPS

In search windows on the Internet:
• Use quotation marks around a phrase to search for that exact combination of words (for example, "universal health care").

• Use the minus sign to eliminate certain words from your search (for instance, health care–private).

• Use a colon and an extension to search a specific site (for example, Medicaid:.gov for all government website mentions of that health care system).

• Use the word Define and a colon to search for word definitions (such as Define: humanitarian).

[Note: health care can be written as one word, healthcare.]

▶ Supporters of universal health care agree that health care is a human right, but have different ideas on how to implement and pay for it. Massachusetts senator and 2020 Democratic presidential candidate Elizabeth Warren, who spoke to this crowd in Boston, believes Medicare for all can be financed through such things as new taxes on corporations.

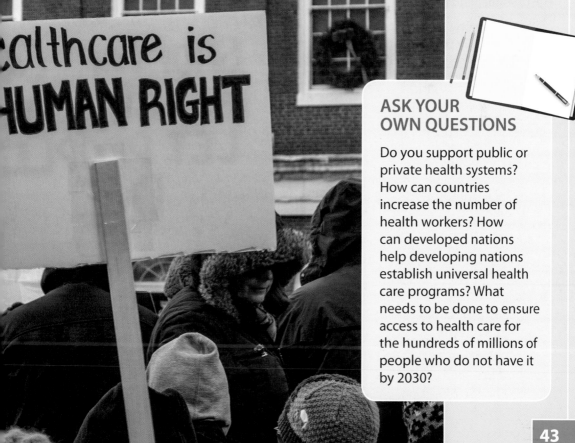

INCREASING COST OF HEALTH CARE DUE TO AGING POPULATION
Based on U.S. figures for 2016

Population aged 60 or over (thousands)

Canada:
- 2017: 23.5% — 8,590
- 2050: 32.0% — 14,368

U.S.A.:
- 2017: 21.5% — 69,774
- 2050: 27.8% — 108,425

U.S.A. Health care costs by age group (spending per capita)

Age group	Spending per capita
0–18	$3,552
19–44	$4,458
45–64	$9,513
65–84	$16,872
85+	$32,411

Canada

U.S.A.

calthcare is HUMAN RIGHT

ASK YOUR OWN QUESTIONS

Do you support public or private health systems? How can countries increase the number of health workers? How can developed nations help developing nations establish universal health care programs? What needs to be done to ensure access to health care for the hundreds of millions of people who do not have it by 2030?

GLOSSARY

administrative Activities related to running a business or organization

advocates People who support or recommend a policy or plan

analyzing Studying carefully

autonomy Being able to self-govern or manage independently

bias Strong feelings for or against something

bibliographies Lists of books referred to in a published work

Bolsheviks Members of the Russian Social Democratic political party that took power in Russia in 1917

campaign A planned set of activities or events intended to achieve a particular social or political goal

censorship The act of suppressing words, images, and ideas that are seen as offensive

contagious A disease or belief that passes easily from one person to another

context The situation in which an event, idea, or statement takes place

credentials Personal qualities or qualifications

credible Trusted, reliable

crowdfunding Raising money online in small amounts through many people

CT scan An X-ray taken to create a detailed image of a body part

economically Related to the business, finance, and resources of a country

equitable Fair and impartial

Great Depression A worldwide economic downturn that lasted from 1929 to 1939

human right A basic right based on shared values that is believed to belong to every person in the world

immunization The act of making someone immune to something, often through vaccination

incentive Something provided as a motivation to do something

income tax A tax levied on personal income

industrialized Having built up a system of industries

lobbyists People who take part in an organized attempt to influence lawmakers

mandatory Required by law

media Types of mass communication such as TV, newspapers, radio, and the Internet. Social media includes blogs, chat lines, text messaging, and online communities for networking.

non-governmental organizations (NGOs) Not-for-profit groups formed on a local, national, or international level that are not run by the government

poverty Extremely poor and not having enough money to pay for basic needs such as shelter, food, and clothing

premiums Sums of money paid to an insurance company for protection or help

prenatal Before birth

prescription Instruction issued by a doctor to allow a patient to be issued with a medicine

publicly funded Paid for out of taxation

reference A source a person can look to for information

regulated Controlled by a rule, standard, or law

resolution Formal expression of opinion or action agreed by a lawmaking body

revolution A sudden and forceful change in government

socialist A person who believes that goods and services are owned and managed by communities. There is no private ownership.

social welfare A group of services meant to provide assistance to people in need

society A large, organized group of people who are linked by their location, religion, culture, or other things

source materials Original documents or other pieces of evidence or key information

statistical Using data compiled in numerical form

subsidized Supported through partial payment

think tanks Groups of experts producing advice and ideas on specific political, social, or economic problems

transcripts Written or printed versions of a speech or broadcast

SOURCE NOTES

QUOTATIONS
p. 4 https://tinyurl.com/yx8og5ww
p. 6 https://tinyurl.com/yyzykhyr
p. 10 https://tinyurl.com/y6x4qml6
p. 22 https://tinyurl.com/y66kb73x
p. 28 https://tinyurl.com/y3zsb9jt
p. 39 https://tinyurl.com/yxl4jzda

REFERENCES USED FOR THIS BOOK

Chapter 1: A Controversial Issue, pages 4–7
https://tinyurl.com/y558hmdf
https://tinyurl.com/y37f9era
https://tinyurl.com/ycju4u4w
https://tinyurl.com/y2cpn3c8
https://tinyurl.com/y5r93rqk
https://tinyurl.com/yysbw9zz

Chapter 2: How to Get Informed, pages 8–13
https://tinyurl.com/yxqr8kkg
https://tinyurl.com/yy3vfw4v
https://tinyurl.com/y4vyxsky
https://tinyurl.com/ybbzjut5
https://tinyurl.com/y4dft5d6

Chapter 3: The Big Picture, pages 14–23
https://tinyurl.com/yyreqj9l
https://tinyurl.com/yxatyvrj
https://tinyurl.com/y3gm3qc3
https://tinyurl.com/yyl9uxkk
https://tinyurl.com/y662g5vj
https://tinyurl.com/y6kupfot
https://tinyurl.com/yxmtkccm
https://tinyurl.com/y3uzzmga
https://tinyurl.com/y5hvhgxv
https://tinyurl.com/yy3wx33n

Chapter 4: Making an Informed Decision, pages 24–35
https://tinyurl.com/y3cspq5z
https://tinyurl.com/y6facvvs
https://tinyurl.com/7bxofbm
https://tinyurl.com/y3mgzfh6
https://tinyurl.com/y2vgdn6q
https://tinyurl.com/y2zr6e3f
https://tinyurl.com/y5z7xg5u
https://tinyurl.com/y3kjsmvq
https://tinyurl.com/ycju4u4w
https://tinyurl.com/y6asm7pn
https://tinyurl.com/yajxwvdz
https://tinyurl.com/y26ws53t

Chapter 5: Staying Informed, pages 36–39
https://tinyurl.com/yyr5cljw
https://tinyurl.com/yxatyvrj
https://tinyurl.com/wwzte7a
https://tinyurl.com/groz64m
https://tinyurl.com/yy96adyd

Chapter 6: Plan of Action, pages 40–43
https://tinyurl.com/y5bbego4
https://tinyurl.com/yyreqj9l
https://tinyurl.com/yy36cwjg

FIND OUT MORE

Finding good source material on the Internet can sometimes be a challenge. When analyzing how reliable the information is, consider these points:

- Who is the author of the page? Is it an expert in the field or a person who experienced the event?

- Is the site well known and up to date? A page that has not been updated for several years probably has out-of-date information.

- Can you verify the facts with another site? Always double-check information.

- Have you checked all possible sites? Don't just look on the first page a search engine provides.

- Remember to try government sites and research papers.

- Have you recorded website addresses and names? Keep this data for a later time so you can backtrack and verify the information you want to use.

WEBSITES

Learn about Universal Health Coverage Day:
http://universalhealthcoverageday.org/about/

Find out more about WHO standards for universal health care:
www.who.int/who-un/about/uhc/en/

Get the facts on the JLN:
www.jointlearningnetwork.org/

Discover the work of the Global Health Network:
https://globalhealth.org/

Learn more about the history of U.S. Medicare and Medicaid:
www.lbjlibrary.org/press/media-kit/medicare-and-medicaid

BOOKS

Forman, Lillian E. *Health Care Reform*. ABDO, 2019.

Green, John. *The Fault in Our Stars*. Penguin Books, 2014.

Jarrow, Gail. *Bubonic Panic: When Plague Invaded America*. Calkins Creek, an Imprint of Highlights, 2016.

Miller, Debra A. *Health Care*. Lucent Books, 2011.

Stevenson, Tyler. *Health Care: Limits, Laws, and Lives at Stake*. Lucent Books, 2018.

ABOUT THE AUTHOR

Heather C. Hudak has written hundreds of children's books on all types of topics. When she is not writing, Heather enjoys traveling all over the world. She also enjoys camping in the mountains near her home with her husband and many rescue dogs and cats.

INDEX